HIGH INTENSITY INTERCOURSE TRAINING

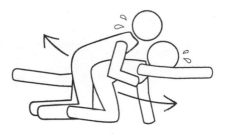

CONTENTS

It's easier to say, 'Screw it, I give up,' than, 'Screw you, let's get started!'

With the **Bench** you must stay firm, keep the core tight and wait for the sperm.

60 Pumps
20 Seconds Rest

Difficulty

Tricky

Intensity

Level 3

CORE EXERCISES

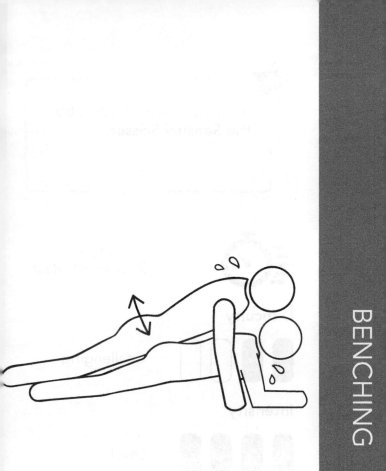

CORE EXERCISES

If the gym doesn't cut it, try the **Sensual Scissor**.

60 Pumps
20 Seconds Rest

Difficulty

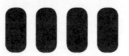

Challenging

Intensity

Level 4

CORE EXERCISES

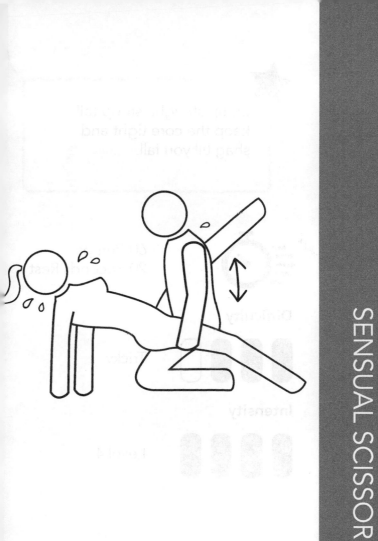

CORE EXERCISES

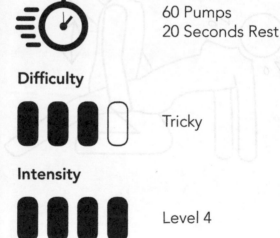

Sit up straight, sit up tall,
keep the core tight and
shag till you fall.

60 Pumps
20 Seconds Rest

Difficulty

Tricky

Intensity

Level 4

HUG HOLD

CORE EXERCISES

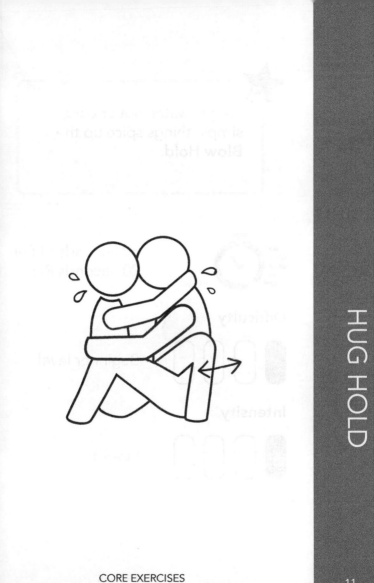

Gargle water, hot or cold, simple things spice up the **Blow Hold**.

60 Seconds of Fun
20 Seconds Rest

Difficulty

Beginner level

Intensity

Level 1

CORE EXERCISES

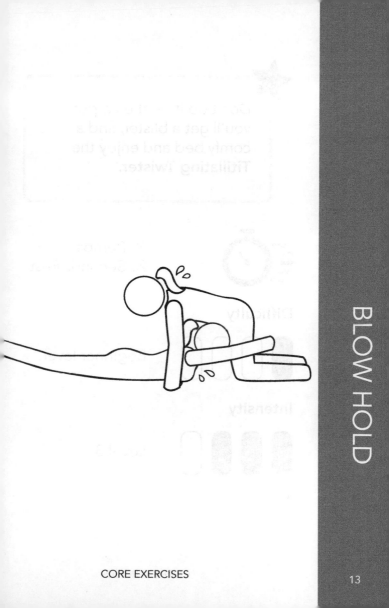

Don't do it on the carpet, you'll get a blister, find a comfy bed and enjoy the **Titillating Twister.**

60 Pumps
20 Seconds Rest

Difficulty

Beginner level

Intensity

Level 3

CORE EXERCISES

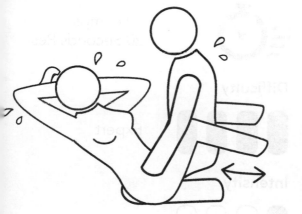

CORE EXERCISES

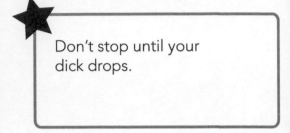

Don't stop until your dick drops.

60 Pumps
20 Seconds Rest

Difficulty

Expert

Intensity

Level 1

CORE EXERCISES

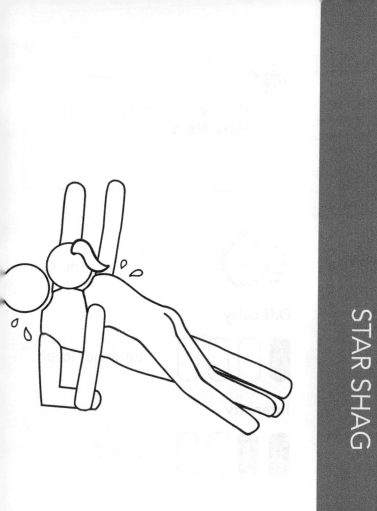

STAR SHAG

Be brave, be bold, hold the **Hard Hold**.

60 Pumps
20 Seconds Rest

Difficulty

Beginner level

Intensity

Level 2

CORE EXERCISES

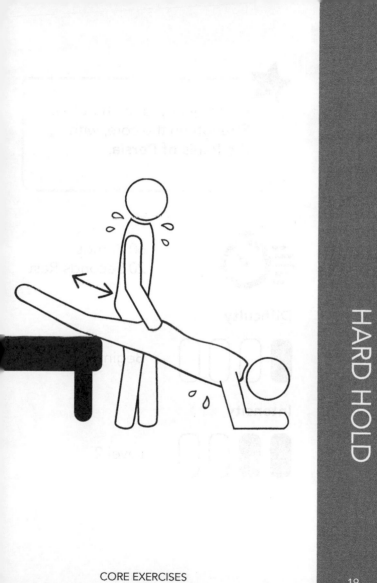

CORE EXERCISES

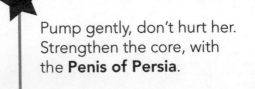

Pump gently, don't hurt her. Strengthen the core, with the **Penis of Persia**.

60 Pumps
20 Seconds Rest

Difficulty

Beginner level

Intensity

Level 2

CORE EXERCISES

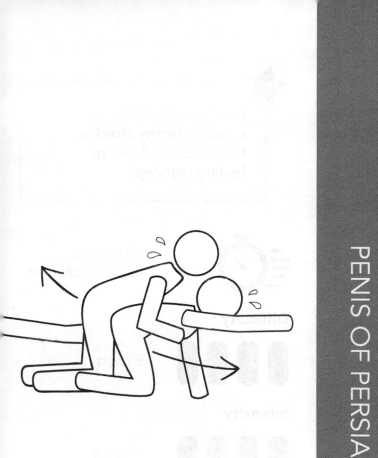

CORE EXERCISES

Randy, horny, tubby or scrawny, **Horny Hold** is the sexercise if you're feeling raunchy.

60 Pumps
20 Seconds Rest

Difficulty

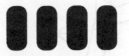

Expert

Intensity

Level 4

CORE EXERCISES

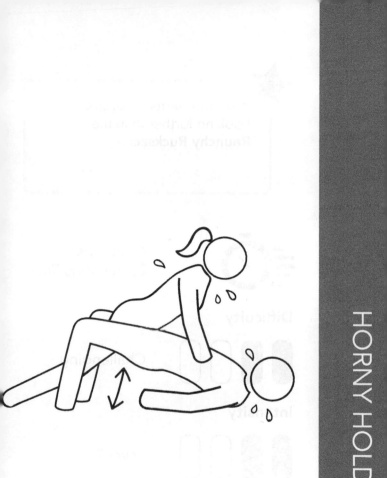

CORE EXERCISES

After the perfect six-pack?
Look no further than the
Raunchy Rucksack.

60 Pumps
20 Seconds Rest

Difficulty

Challenging

Intensity

Level 2

CORE EXERCISES

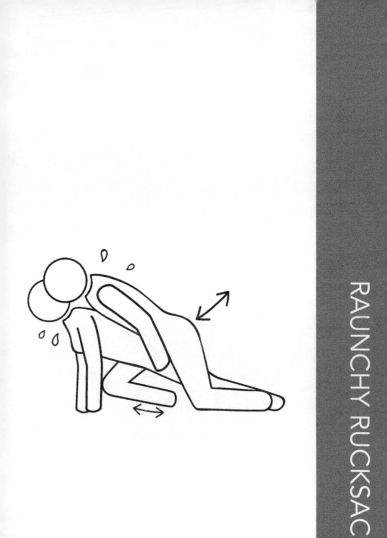

CORE EXERCISES

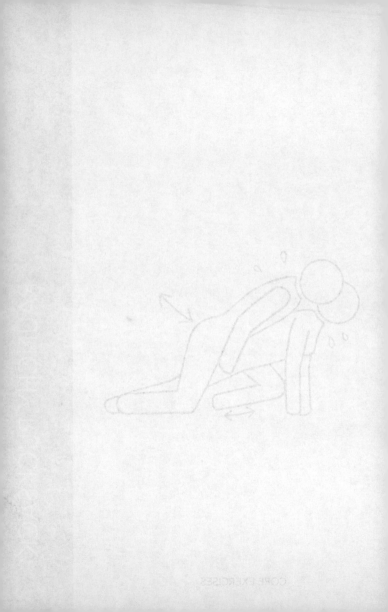

'Sex insane or remain the same.'

Bend and blow, build a strong back and let the semen flow.

60 Pumps
20 Seconds Rest

Difficulty

Tricky

Intensity

Level 1

BENDY BLOWY

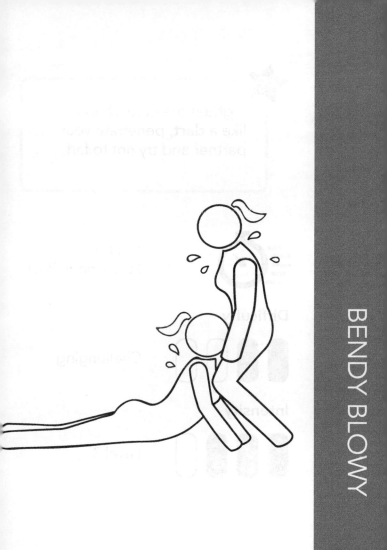

BACK EXERCISES

Tighten the core, shape like a **dart**, penetrate your partner and try not to fart.

60 Pumps
20 Seconds Rest

Difficulty

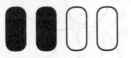

Chellenging

Intensity

Level 3

BACK EXERCISES

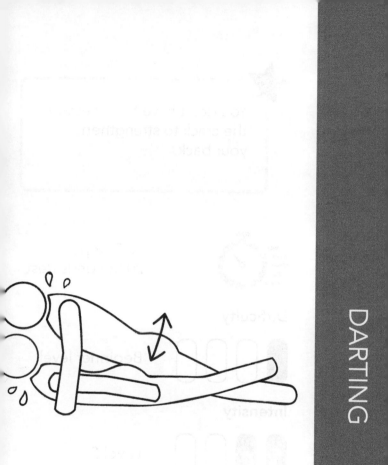

BACK EXERCISES

You don't have to penetrate the crack to strengthen your back.

60 Pumps
20 Seconds Rest

Difficulty

Beginner level

Intensity

Level 2

PLANK WANK

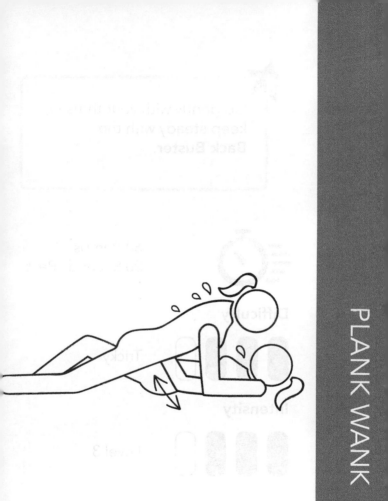

BACK EXERCISES

Go gently with your thruster, keep steady with the **Back Buster**.

60 Pumps
20 Seconds Rest

Difficulty

Tricky

Intensity

Level 3

BACK BUSTER

BACK EXERCISES

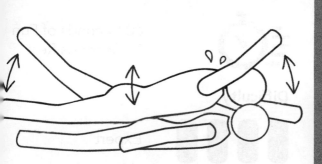

BACK BUSTER

Don't panic, if he's well hung, keep your back straight and work the tongue.

60 Seconds of Fun
20 Seconds Rest

Difficulty

Expert

Intensity

Level 2

TONGUE TWISTER

BACK EXERCISES

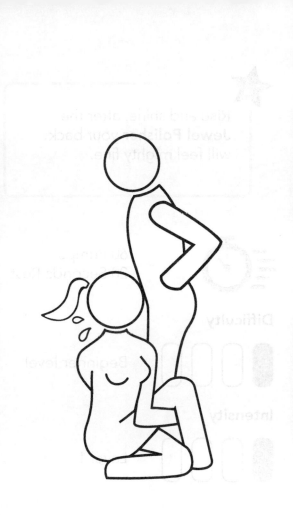

BACK EXERCISES

Rise and shine, after the **Jewel Polisher** your back will feel mighty fine.

60 Pumps
20 Seconds Rest

Difficulty

Beginner level

Intensity

Level 1

BACK EXERCISES

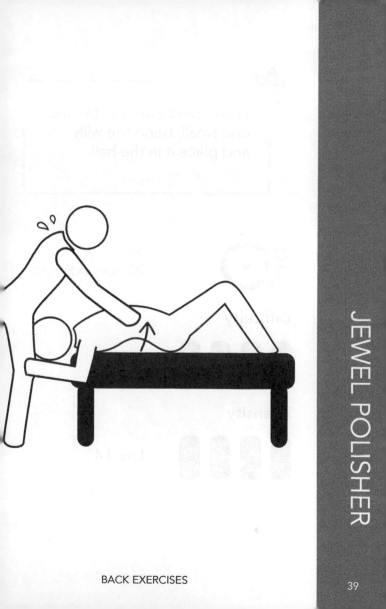

BACK EXERCISES

Works best with one tall and one small, bend the willy and place it in the hall.

60 Pumps
20 Seconds Rest

Difficulty

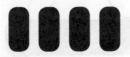

Expert

Intensity

Level 4

BRIDGE SUPPORT

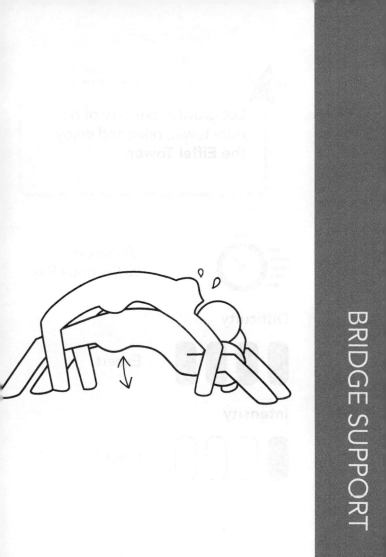

Let gravity take care of his mini tower, relax and enjoy the **Eiffel Tower**.

60 Pumps
20 Seconds Rest

Difficulty

Expert

Intensity

Level 1

EIFFEL TOWER

BACK EXERCISES

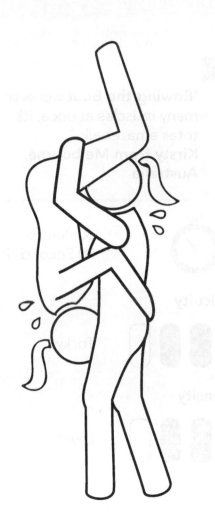

'**Rowing the Boat** works so many muscles at once, it's totes amazeballs.'
Kirsty from Melbourne, Australia

60 Pumps
20 Seconds Rest

Difficulty

Tricky

Intensity

Level 3

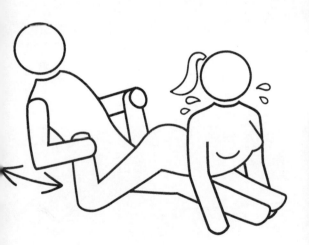

ROW THE BOAT

BACK EXERCISES

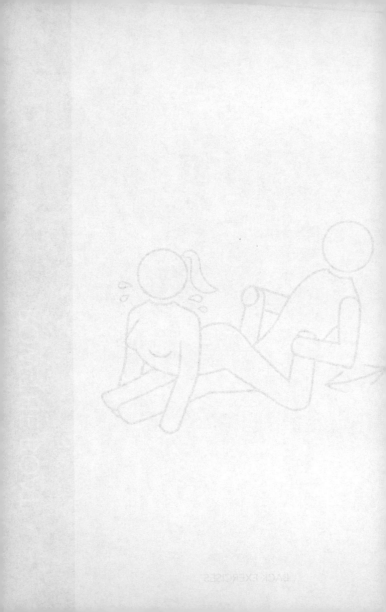

'Have sex today, your future self will thank you for it tomorrow.'

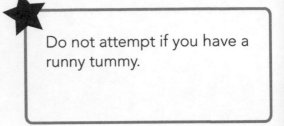

Do not attempt if you have a runny tummy.

60 Pumps
20 Seconds Rest

SPIDER RIDER

Difficulty

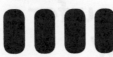

Expert

Intensity

Level 4

LEG EXERCISES

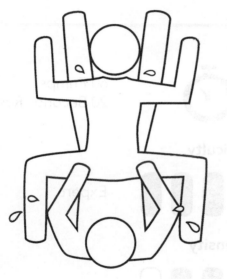

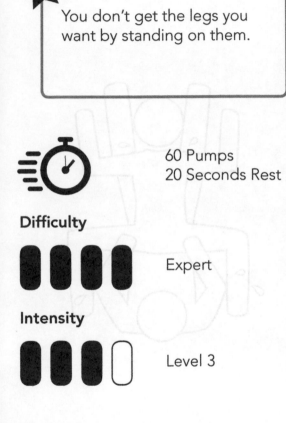

You don't get the legs you want by standing on them.

60 Pumps
20 Seconds Rest

Difficulty

Expert

Intensity

Level 3

SPLIT AND DIP

LEG EXERCISES

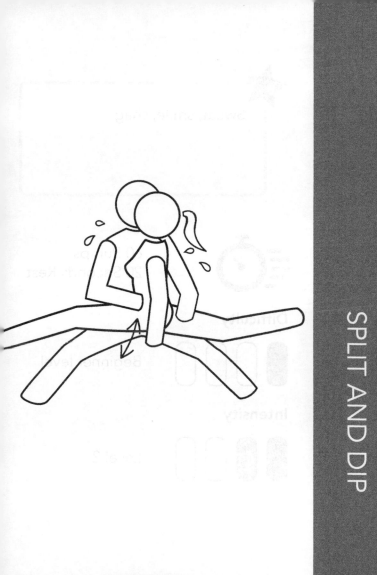

LEG EXERCISES

Sweat, smile, shag.

60 Pumps
20 Seconds Rest

Difficulty

Beginner level

Intensity

Level 2

LEG EXERCISES

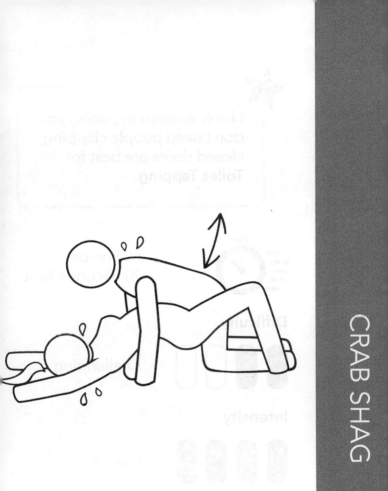

Never attempt in public, you don't need people clapping, closed doors are best for **Toilet Tapping**.

60 Pumps
20 Seconds Rest

Difficulty

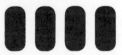

Challenging

Intensity

Level 4

LEG EXERCISES

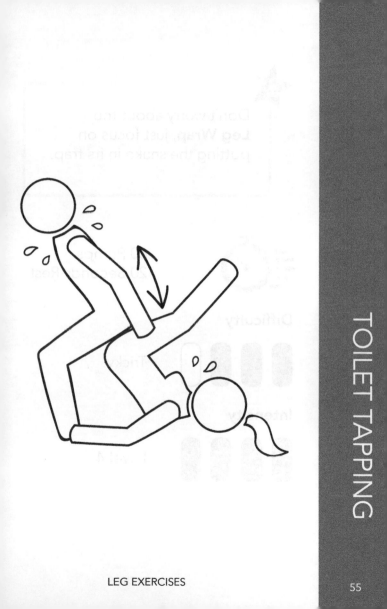

LEG EXERCISES

Don't worry about the **Leg Wrap**, just focus on putting the snake in its trap.

60 Pumps
20 Seconds Rest

Difficulty

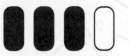

Tricky

Intensity

Level 4

LEG WRAP

LEG EXERCISES

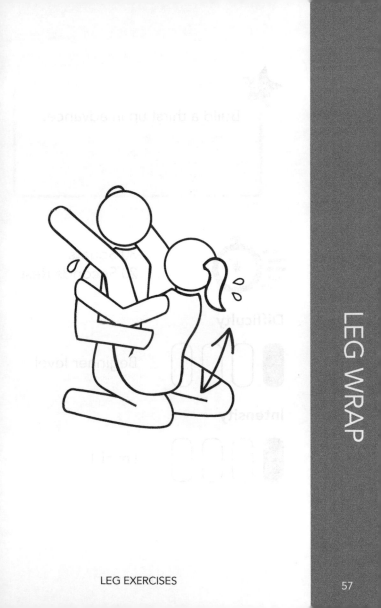

Build a thirst up in advance.

30 Squats
20 Seconds Rest

Difficulty

Beginner level

Intensity

Level 1

SQUAT SQUIRTS

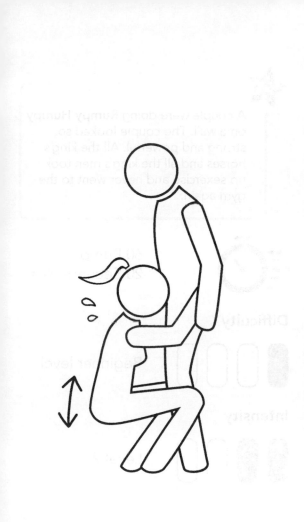

SQUAT SQUIRTS

A couple were doing **Rumpy Humpy** on a wall. The couple looked so strong and powerful. All the king's horses and all the king's men took up sexercise and never went to the gym again.

60 Pumps
20 Seconds Rest

Difficulty

Beginner level

Intensity

Level 2

RUMPY HUMPY

LEG EXERCISES

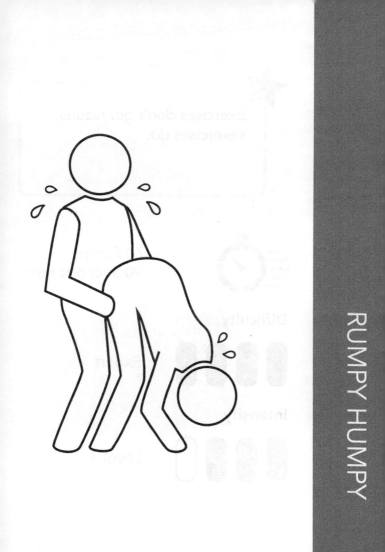

LEG EXERCISES

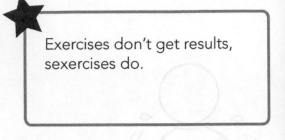

> Exercises don't get results, sexercises do.

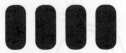

60 Pumps
20 Seconds Rest

Difficulty

Expert

Intensity

Level 3

QUAD BURN BANG

LEG EXERCISES

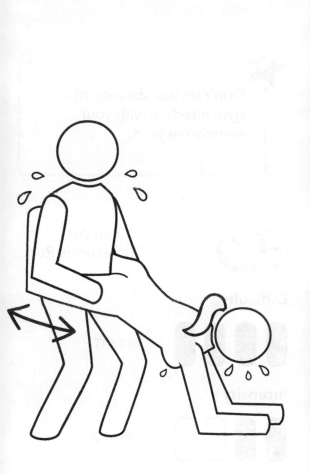

QUAD BURN BANG

Don't let the absence of a gym interfere with your exercise regime.

40 Pumps
20 Seconds Rest

Difficulty

Expert

Intensity

Level 2

SCISSOR SET

LEG EXERCISES

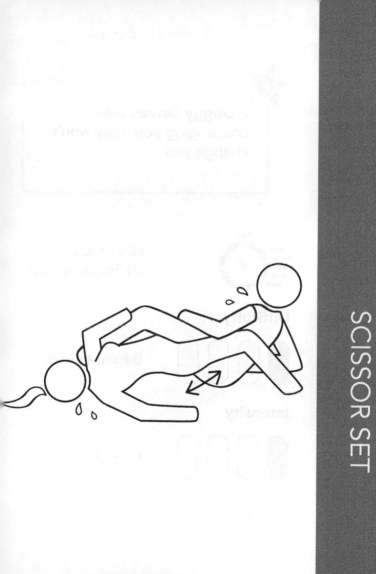

LEG EXERCISES

If **Doggy Drives** aren't challenging you, they won't change you.

60 Pumps
20 Seconds Rest

Difficulty

Beginner level

Intensity

Level 1

LEG EXERCISES

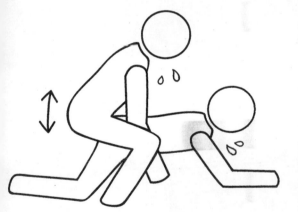

LEG EXERCISES

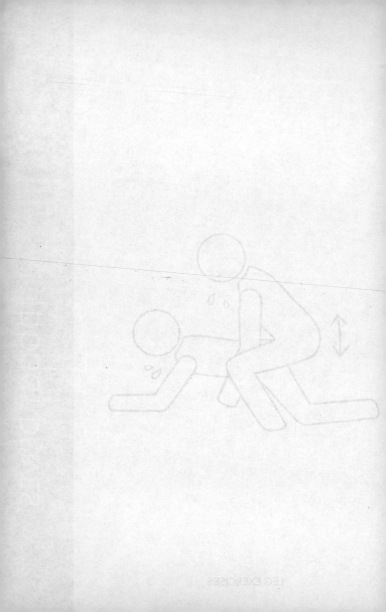

'Don't wish for
a good body,
shag for it.'

X marks the G-spot, now shag till your knees drop.

60 Pumps
20 Seconds Rest

Difficulty

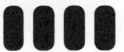

Expert

Intensity

Level 4

X REP

GLUTE EXERCISES

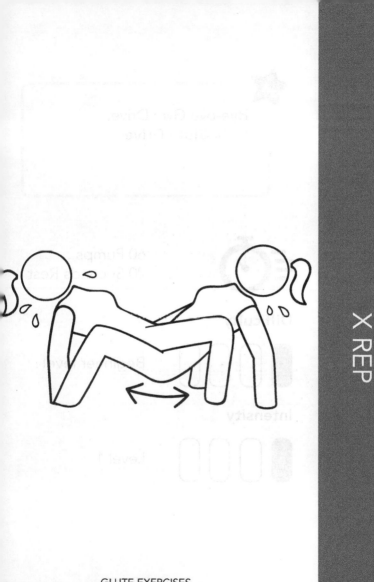

GLUTE EXERCISES

> Bye-bye Gym Drive.
> Hi-hi **Glute Drive**.

60 Pumps
20 Seconds Rest

Difficulty

Beginner level

Intensity

Level 1

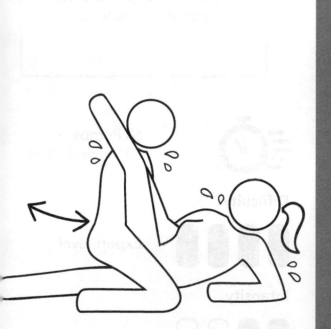

GLUTE EXERCISES

Try out the **Pony Bounces**,
and shed a few ounces.

60 Pumps
20 Seconds Rest

Difficulty

Expert level

Intensity

Level 2

GLUTE EXERCISES

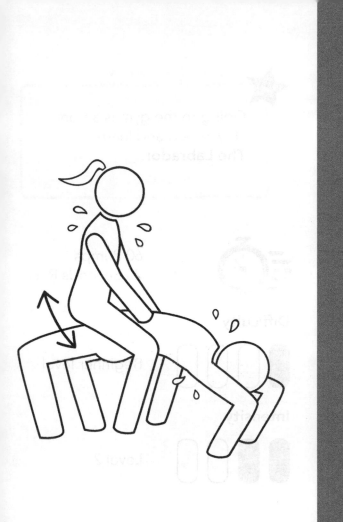

GLUTE EXERCISES

Going to the gym is a bore, stay in bed and learn **The Labrador**.

60 Pumps
20 Seconds Rest

Difficulty

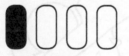

Beginner level

Intensity

Level 2

GLUTE EXERCISES

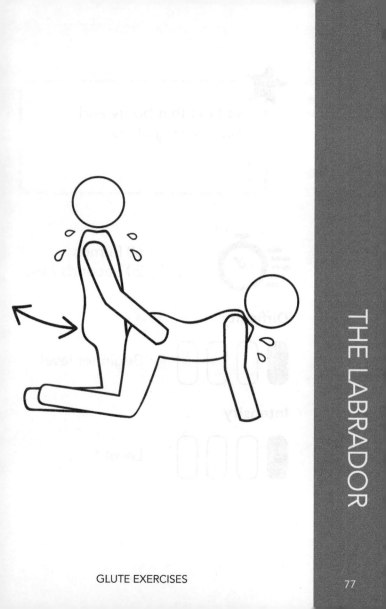

GLUTE EXERCISES

Sort out that booty and work those gluteys.

60 Pumps
20 Seconds Rest

Difficulty

Beginner level

Intensity

Level 1

GLUTE EXERCISES

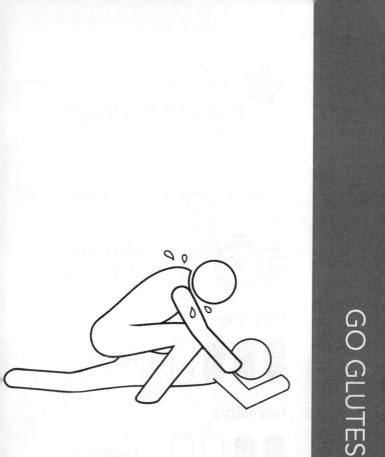

GLUTE EXERCISES

Only one **Bridge Bang** from your destination.

60 Pumps
20 Seconds Rest

Difficulty

Tricky

Intensity

Level 2

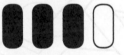

BRIDGE BANG

GLUTE EXERCISES

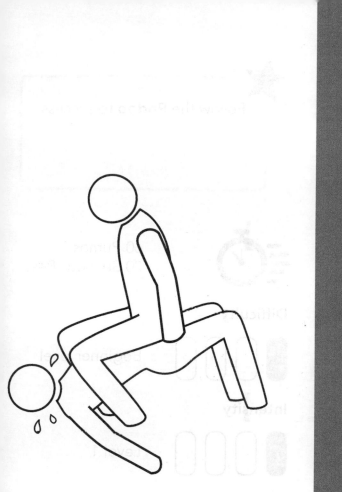

BRIDGE BANG

Follow the **Rodeo** to success.

60 Pumps
20 Seconds Rest

Difficulty

Beginner level

Intensity

Level 1

GLUTE EXERCISES

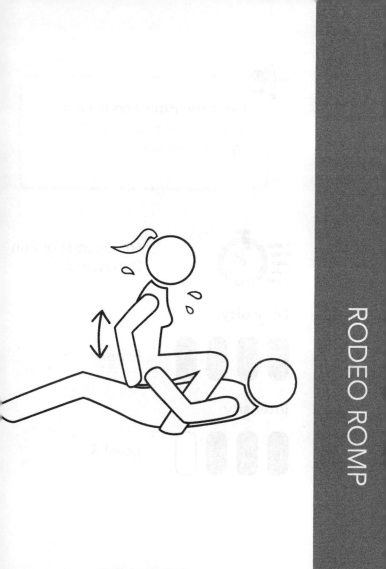

GLUTE EXERCISES

Light the **Pipe** and have a smoke, just make sure he's a hygienic bloke.

60 Seconds of Fun
20 Seconds Rest

Difficulty

Expert

Intensity

Level 3

GLUTE EXERCISES

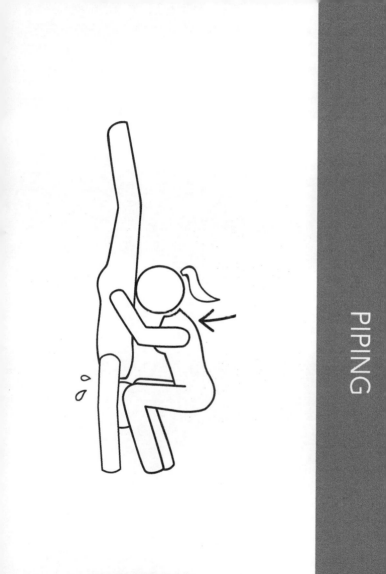

GLUTE EXERCISES

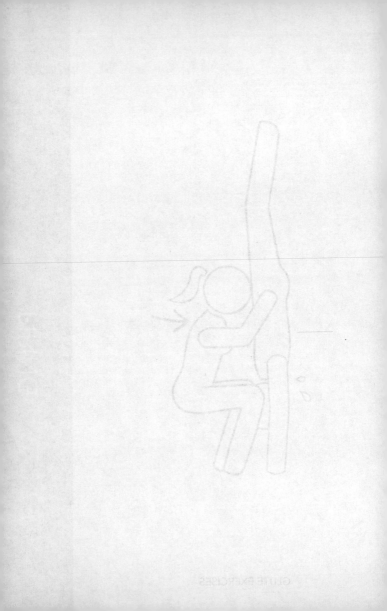

'The shagging you do today will be the strength you feel tomorrow.'

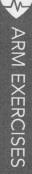

> Don't wait, start now,
> burn the bingos and
> **Milk the Cow.**

45 Shakes
20 Seconds Rest

Difficulty

Beginner level

Intensity

Level 1

ARM EXERCISES

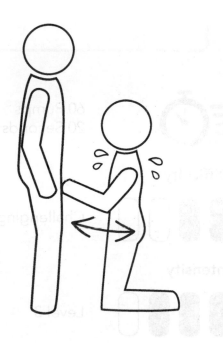

MILKING THE COW

Rise up, tickle the tip, have fun with the **Dick Dips**.

60 Pumps
20 Seconds Rest

Difficulty

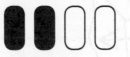

Challenging

Intensity

Level 3

DICK DIPS

ARM EXERCISES

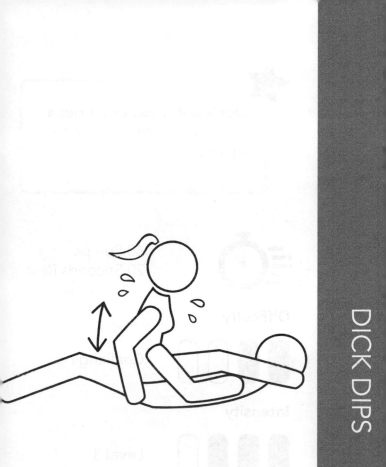

ARM EXERCISES

Don't worry, you won't get a ticket, to enhance pleasure, try and flick it.

60 Pumps
20 Seconds Rest

Difficulty

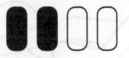

Challenging

Intensity

Level 3

REVERSE PARK

ARM EXERCISES

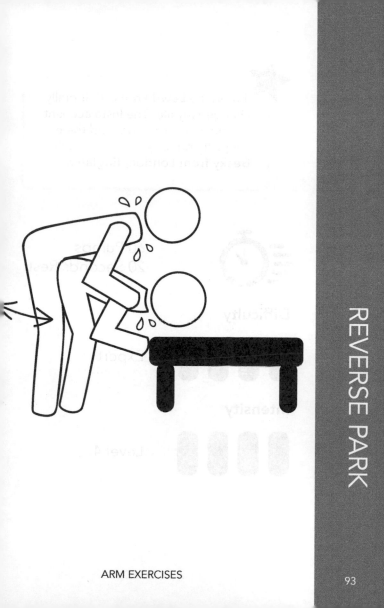

REVERSE PARK

LEWD LOTUS

> 'I tried the **Lewd Lotus**, it's literally changed my life. The Insta account has doubled overnight and the ex keeps trying to get back in touch.'
> **Becky from London, England**

60 Pumps
20 Seconds Rest

Difficulty

Expert

Intensity

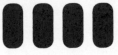

Level 4

ARM EXERCISES

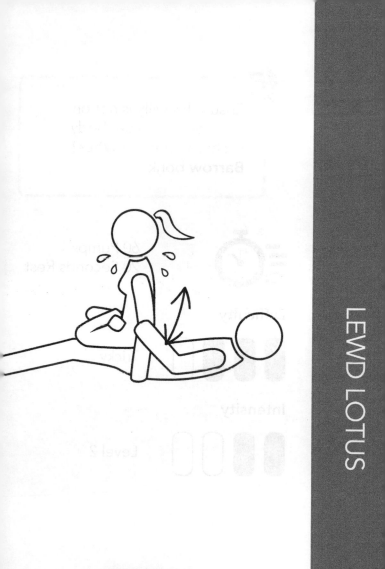

ARM EXERCISES

Ensure his willy is not on the wonk, get your body in shape with the **Wheel Barrow** bonk.

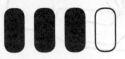

60 Pumps
20 Seconds Rest

Difficulty

Tricky

Intensity

Level 2

WHEEL BARROW

ARM EXERCISES

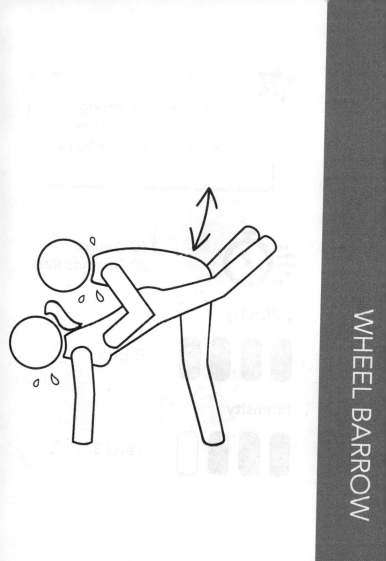

WHEEL BARROW

Upside down, the wrong way round, it's always fun with the **Headstand Pound**.

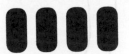

60 Pumps
20 Seconds Rest

Difficulty

Expert

Intensity

Level 3

ARM EXERCISES

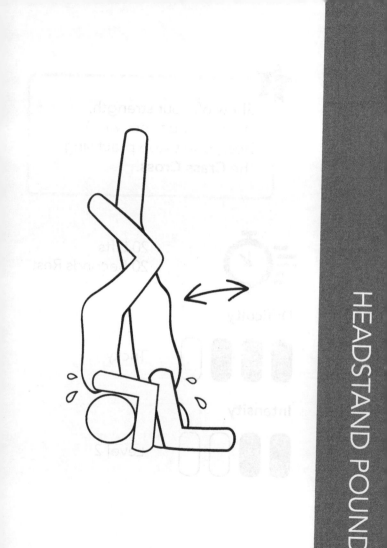

HEADSTAND POUND

Show off your strength, show your partner who's boss, don't stop practising the **Crass Cross**.

20 Lifts
20 Seconds Rest

Difficulty

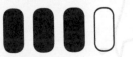

Tricky

Intensity

Level 2

ARM EXERCISES

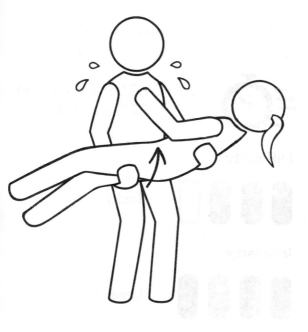

ARM EXERCISES

Avoid doing this position in January when extra weight is a disadvantage.

60 Pumps
20 Seconds Rest

Difficulty

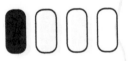

Beginner level

Intensity

Level 2

ARM EXERCISES

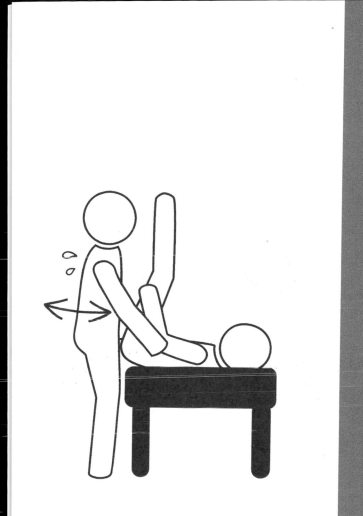

ARM EXERCISES

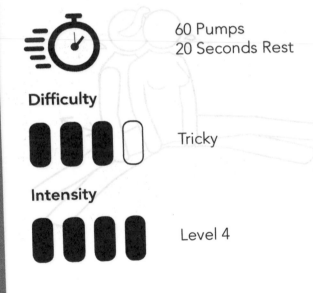

Ready steady, start on cue,
enjoy your exercise with a
Moon View.

60 Pumps
20 Seconds Rest

Difficulty

Tricky

Intensity

Level 4

MOON VIEW

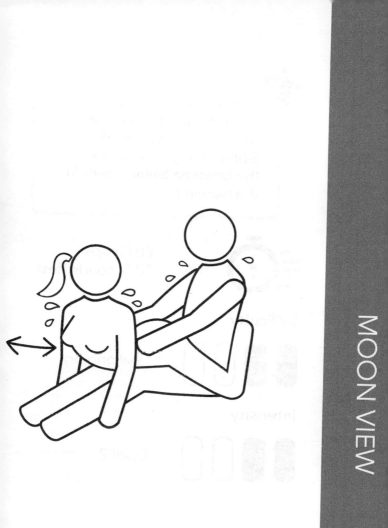

CARDIO EXERCISES

> Start your sexercise with the **Drunken Sailor**, start your sexercise with the **Drunken Sailor**, start your sexercise with the **Drunken Sailor**… early in the morning.

60 Pumps
20 Seconds Rest

Difficulty

Challenging

Intensity

Level 2

CARDIO EXERCISES

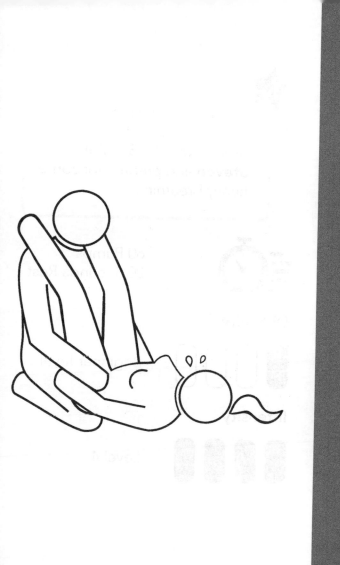

CARDIO EXERCISES

If you're not feeling adventurous or at all pretentious, try **Sensible Steven** and prepare for some heavy breathin'.

60 Pumps
20 Seconds Rest

Difficulty

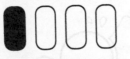

Beginner level

Intensity

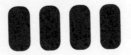

Level 4

CARDIO EXERCISES

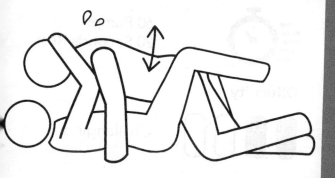

CARDIO EXERCISES

Ride hard, ride fast, ride
until you both orgasm and
finish top of the class.

60 Pumps
20 Seconds Rest

Difficulty

Challenging

Intensity

Level 4

CARDIO EXERCISES

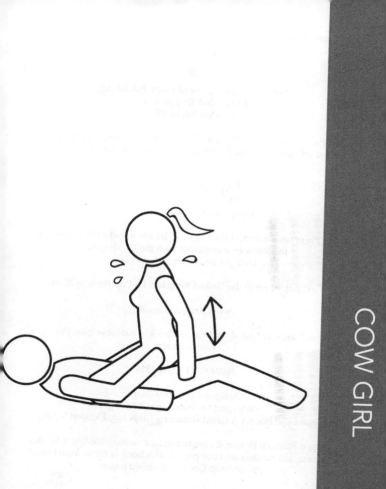

CARDIO EXERCISES

21

Pop Press, an imprint of Ebury Publishing,
20 Vauxhall Bridge Road,
London SW1V 2SA

Pop Press is part of the Penguin Random House group of companies
whose addresses can be found at global.penguinrandomhouse.com

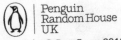

Penguin
Random House
UK

Pop Press have asserted their right to be identified as the author of
this Work in accordance with the Copyright,
Designs and Patents Act 1988

First published in the United Kingdom by Pop Press in 2018

www.penguin.co.uk

A CIP catalogue record for this book is available from the
British Library

ISBN 9781529102819

Designed by Emily Snape
Packaged by Saturday Publishing
Printed and bound in Great Britain by Clays Ltd, Elcograf S.p.A.

Penguin Random House is committed to a sustainable future for our
business, our readers and our planet. This book is made from Forest
Stewardship Council® certified paper.

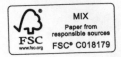